ADHD

Medication and Symptom Tracking Journal for Adults

Right Track Publishing

Olathe, Kansas

ADHD Medication and Symptom Tracking Journal for Adults

Revised and Updated Edition

Right Track Publishing
P.O. Box 4712, Olathe, KS 66063
www.righttrackpublishing.com
Printed in the United States of America
ISBN: 978-1-947037-10-6

PSYCHOLOGY / Psychopathology / Attention-Deficit Disorder
REFERENCE / Personal & Practical Guides

How to Use This Journal

If you've been recently diagnosed with Attention Deficit Hyperactivity Disorder and started taking medication, keeping a journal can help!

It often takes weeks (or months) for you and your doctor to know which medication and what dose is best in alleviating the challenging symptoms that adults with ADHD live with day to day. By keeping track of medication type, side effects (if any), and symptom relief, you and your doctor can make necessary adjustments in your treatment plan.

This journal allows you to keep track of your medication and symptom management for ADHD for 90 days. Each day includes two fill-in-the-blank pages. Use this for your personal records or to assist your doctor in deciding his treatment plan.

If you skip or miss a dose, be sure to still answer the questions on the "symptom" page of that day. Doing so will give you a clearer picture of how well your symptoms are being managed with or without medication.

The back of the journal has blank pages for you to keep extra notes, write about your experiences or feelings, and any other significant observations.

You might not have some of the symptoms listed. Each person with ADHD has their own unique set of symptoms and challenges. It depends on the severity of the condition (mild, moderate, or severe) and your subtype: Inattentive, Hyperactive, or Combination.

Medication Details

Date ____________ ____________ Day of Week

Medication ____________ Dosage __________

Skipped Medication Yes No

Time(s) medication taken:

AM __________ AM __________
PM __________ PM __________

Time(s) medication wore off: ________ ________

Taken: [1] [2] On empty stomach
[1] [2] With Food

Kind of food __________________________________

____

Appetite: Poor Average Good

Slept from ________ to ________ Total: _______

Felt rested after waking: Yes No

Side Effects: __________________________________

____

____

____

____

No dejaban de tener razón Ogden y Richards, en consecuencia, cuando señalaban que la relación entre referente y referencia (a esta última ahora la sustituyo por "concepto") no es fija, sino sólo *adecuada* y que no es una sola, sino tan múltiple como lo determinen los contextos en los que se forma. En cambio, lo que no tomaban en cuenta es el papel del signo (o "símbolo") en la propia formación del concepto. Lo que permiten demostrar la teoría piagetiana y la lingüística es que el signo no se *asocia* posteriormente al concepto previamente formado o al referente, sino que se *disocia* de ellos en el proceso de formación tanto del esquema cognoscitivo como del mismo signo. Es la disociación tanto del esquema como del signo respecto de la experiencia de los objetos la que define la inteligencia humana (puesto que el resto de los animales la logran en una medida muy limitada, si acaso) y la que vuelve tan poderosas a las lenguas.

La relación entre el signo disociado de los objetos en cuyo contexto pragmático se produjo y el o los esquemas cognoscitivos con los cuales se formó y a los cuales contribuyó a formar se vuelve problemática, precisamente porque no es la de una simple etiqueta de las cosas o de los conceptos, sino una entidad significativa que, por su propia naturaleza cognoscitiva y lingüística, queda siempre en la posibilidad de recrear ideas de los objetos o de recrear conceptos. Si el signo fuera un mero soporte material de la referencia, una etiqueta o un nombre de las cosas, su capacidad significativa no rebasaría las posibilidades de los lenguajes de señales marítimas o de las señales de tráfico.

Es precisamente por esto por lo que se plantea el conflicto con el que comencé este trabajo: cómo es posible que un signo —un término, en el caso que nos interesa— cumpla con las condiciones analíticas necesarias y suficientes como para corresponder unívoca y verdaderamente al objeto a que se refiere. La libertad significativa que conlleva el signo por su propia naturaleza complica el discurso veritativo, que es el que interesa al filósofo, al lógico, al científico, al técnico y… a muchos terminólogos.

La construcción del término

Conviene entonces reconstruir el problema planteado por Putnam en términos de lo argumentado:

> (1) El hecho de que el *concepto* 'clase natural, la totalidad de cuyos miembros vive bajo el agua, respira por agallas, etc.' no se ajuste estrictamente al *significado de la palabra Fish*, no quiere decir que el concepto no *corresponda* al conjunto de los animales acuáticos significados por la *palabra Fish*, ni que el *significado de la palabra Fish* deba considerarse exactamente correspondiente a las características reales de esos animales. […] el *concepto* no es exacta-

Symptom Details

Rate the following on a scale of 1 to 5:
(1-Poor 2- Meh 3- Decent 4- Good 5-Super)

Mood _____ Focus _____ Memory _____

Energy _____ Motivation _____ Finishing Tasks _____

Patience _____ Impulsivity _____ Restlessness _____

Time Management _____ Emotion Management _____

Other: _____________ _____ _____________ ____

Medication helped today: Yes No Somewhat

Today's Successes: ______________________________

____

____

____

____

Areas for Improvement: __________________________

____

____

____

Rating for This Day
1- Awful / 5- Great

☆☆☆☆☆

Medication Details

Date ____________ ____________ Day of Week

Medication ____________ Dosage __________

Skipped Medication Yes No

Time(s) medication taken:

AM __________ AM __________
PM __________ PM __________

Time(s) medication wore off: ________ ________

Taken: ☐1 ☐2 On empty stomach
☐1 ☐2 With Food

Kind of food ____________________________________

____

Appetite: Poor Average Good

Slept from ________ to _________ Total: _______

Felt rested after waking: Yes No

Side Effects: ____________________________________

____

____

____

____

Symptom Details

Rate the following on a scale of 1 to 5:
(1-Poor 2- Meh 3- Decent 4- Good 5-Super)

Mood _____ Focus _____ Memory _____

Energy _____ Motivation _____ Finishing Tasks _____

Patience _____ Impulsivity _____ Restlessness _____

Time Management _____ Emotion Management _____

Other: _______________ _____ _______________ ____

Medication helped today: Yes No Somewhat

Today's Successes: _______________________________

____

____

____

____

Areas for Improvement: ___________________________

____

____

____

Rating for This Day
1- Awful / 5- Great

☆☆☆☆☆

Medication Details

Date ____________ ____________ Day of Week

Medication ____________ Dosage __________

Skipped Medication Yes No

Time(s) medication taken:

AM __________ AM __________
PM __________ PM __________

Time(s) medication wore off: ________ ________

Taken: ☐1 ☐2 On empty stomach
☐1 ☐2 With Food

Kind of food ______________________________

____

Appetite: Poor Average Good

Slept from ________ to _________ Total: ______

Felt rested after waking: Yes No

Side Effects: _____________________________

____

____

____

____

Symptom Details

Rate the following on a scale of 1 to 5:
(1-Poor 2- Meh 3- Decent 4- Good 5-Super)

Mood _____ Focus _____ Memory _____

Energy _____ Motivation _____ Finishing Tasks _____

Patience _____ Impulsivity _____ Restlessness _____

Time Management _____ Emotion Management _____

Other: ______________ _____ ________________ ____

Medication helped today: Yes No Somewhat

Today's Successes: ________________________________

____

____

____

____

Areas for Improvement: __________________________

____

____

____

Rating for This Day
1- Awful / 5- Great

☆☆☆☆☆

Medication Details

Date ____________ ____________ Day of Week

Medication ____________ Dosage __________

Skipped Medication Yes No

Time(s) medication taken:

AM __________ AM __________
PM __________ PM __________

Time(s) medication wore off: ________ ________

Taken: ☐ 1 ☐ 2 On empty stomach
☐ 1 ☐ 2 With Food

Kind of food ________________________________

____

Appetite: Poor Average Good

Slept from ________ to _________ Total: _______

Felt rested after waking: Yes No

Side Effects: ______________________________

____

____

____

____

Medication Details

Date ___________ ___________ Day of Week

Medication ___________ Dosage _________

Skipped Medication Yes No

Time(s) medication taken:

AM _________ AM _________
PM _________ PM _________

Time(s) medication wore off: _______ _______

Taken: [1] [2] On empty stomach
[1] [2] With Food

Kind of food _______________________________

____

Appetite: Poor Average Good

Slept from _______ to ________ Total: ______

Felt rested after waking: Yes No

Side Effects: _________________________________

____

____

____

____

Symptom Details

Rate the following on a scale of 1 to 5:
(1-Poor 2- Meh 3- Decent 4- Good 5-Super)

Mood _____ Focus _____ Memory _____

Energy _____ Motivation _____ Finishing Tasks _____

Patience _____ Impulsivity _____ Restlessness _____

Time Management _____ Emotion Management _____

Other: ______________ _____ ________________ ____

Medication helped today: Yes No Somewhat

Today's Successes: ______________________________

____

____

____

____

Areas for Improvement: __________________________

____

____

____

Rating for This Day
1- Awful / 5- Great

☆☆☆☆☆

Medication Details

Date ____________ ____________ Day of Week

Medication ____________ Dosage __________

Skipped Medication Yes No

Time(s) medication taken:

AM __________ AM __________
PM __________ PM __________

Time(s) medication wore off: ________ ________

Taken: ☐ 1 ☐ 2 On empty stomach
☐ 1 ☐ 2 With Food

Kind of food __________________________________

____

Appetite: Poor Average Good

Slept from ________ to _________ Total: _______

Felt rested after waking: Yes No

Side Effects: ____________________________________

____

____

____

____

Symptom Details

Rate the following on a scale of 1 to 5:
(1-Poor 2- Meh 3- Decent 4- Good 5-Super)

Mood _____ Focus _____ Memory _____

Energy _____ Motivation _____ Finishing Tasks _____

Patience _____ Impulsivity _____ Restlessness _____

Time Management _____ Emotion Management _____

Other: ______________ _____ ______________ ____

Medication helped today: Yes No Somewhat

Today's Successes: ______________________________

____

____

____

____

Areas for Improvement: __________________________

____

____

____

Rating for This Day
1- Awful / 5- Great

☆☆☆☆☆

Medication Details

Date ____________ ____________ Day of Week

Medication ____________ Dosage __________

Skipped Medication Yes No

Time(s) medication taken:

AM __________ AM __________
PM __________ PM __________

Time(s) medication wore off: ________ ________

Taken: [1] [2] On empty stomach
[1] [2] With Food

Kind of food ___________________________________

____

Appetite: Poor Average Good

Slept from _______ to ________ Total: ______

Felt rested after waking: Yes No

Side Effects: ___________________________________

____

____

____

____

Symptom Details

Rate the following on a scale of 1 to 5:
(1-Poor 2- Meh 3- Decent 4- Good 5-Super)

Mood _____ Focus _____ Memory _____

Energy _____ Motivation _____ Finishing Tasks _____

Patience _____ Impulsivity _____ Restlessness _____

Time Management _____ Emotion Management _____

Other: _______________ _____ _________________ ____

Medication helped today: Yes No Somewhat

Today's Successes: ________________________________

____

____

____

____

Areas for Improvement: ___________________________

____

____

____

Rating for This Day
1- Awful / 5- Great

☆☆☆☆☆

Medication Details

Date ____________ ____________ Day of Week

Medication ____________ Dosage __________

Skipped Medication Yes No

Time(s) medication taken:

AM __________ AM __________
PM __________ PM __________

Time(s) medication wore off: ________ ________

Taken: [1] [2] On empty stomach
[1] [2] With Food

Kind of food ____

____

Appetite: Poor Average Good

Slept from ________ to _________ Total: _______

Felt rested after waking: Yes No

Side Effects: ____

____

____

____

____

Symptom Details

Rate the following on a scale of 1 to 5:
(1-Poor 2- Meh 3- Decent 4- Good 5-Super)

Mood _____ Focus _____ Memory _____

Energy _____ Motivation _____ Finishing Tasks _____

Patience _____ Impulsivity _____ Restlessness _____

Time Management _____ Emotion Management _____

Other: ______________ _____ ________________ ____

Medication helped today: Yes No Somewhat

Today's Successes: ________________________________

____

____

____

____

Areas for Improvement: __________________________

____

____

____

Rating for This Day
1- Awful / 5- Great

☆☆☆☆☆

Symptom Details

Rate the following on a scale of 1 to 5:
(1-Poor 2- Meh 3- Decent 4- Good 5-Super)

Mood _____ Focus _____ Memory _____

Energy _____ Motivation _____ Finishing Tasks _____

Patience _____ Impulsivity _____ Restlessness _____

Time Management _____ Emotion Management _____

Other: _______________ _____ _______________ ____

Medication helped today: Yes No Somewhat

Today's Successes: ______________________________

____

____

____

____

Areas for Improvement: __________________________

____

____

____

Rating for This Day
1- Awful / 5- Great

☆ ☆ ☆ ☆ ☆

Medication Details

Date ______________ ______________ Day of Week

Medication ______________ Dosage ___________

Skipped Medication Yes No

Time(s) medication taken:

AM ___________ AM ___________
PM ___________ PM ___________

Time(s) medication wore off: _________ _________

Taken: ☐1 ☐2 On empty stomach
☐1 ☐2 With Food

Kind of food ____

____

Appetite: Poor Average Good

Slept from _________ to __________ Total: _______

Felt rested after waking: Yes No

Side Effects: ____

____

____

____

____

Symptom Details

Rate the following on a scale of 1 to 5:
(1-Poor 2- Meh 3- Decent 4- Good 5-Super)

Mood _____ Focus _____ Memory _____

Energy _____ Motivation _____ Finishing Tasks _____

Patience _____ Impulsivity _____ Restlessness _____

Time Management _____ Emotion Management _____

Other: _______________ _____ _________________ ____

Medication helped today: Yes No Somewhat

Today's Successes: __________________________________

____

____

____

____

Areas for Improvement: ____________________________

____

____

____

Rating for This Day
1- Awful / 5- Great

☆☆☆☆☆

Medication Details

Date ______________ ______________ Day of Week

Medication ______________ Dosage ___________

Skipped Medication Yes No

Time(s) medication taken:

AM ___________ AM ___________
PM ___________ PM ___________

Time(s) medication wore off: ________ ________

Taken: [1] [2] On empty stomach
[1] [2] With Food

Kind of food ______________________________________

____

Appetite: Poor Average Good

Slept from ________ to _________ Total: _______

Felt rested after waking: Yes No

Side Effects: _______________________________________

____

____

____

____

Symptom Details

Rate the following on a scale of 1 to 5:
(1-Poor 2- Meh 3- Decent 4- Good 5-Super)

Mood _____ Focus _____ Memory _____

Energy _____ Motivation _____ Finishing Tasks _____

Patience _____ Impulsivity _____ Restlessness _____

Time Management _____ Emotion Management _____

Other: _______________ _____ _______________ _____

Medication helped today: Yes No Somewhat

Today's Successes: ____________________________________

____

____

____

____

Areas for Improvement: ____________________________

____

____

____

Rating for This Day
1- Awful / 5- Great

☆☆☆☆☆

Medication Details

Date ____________ ____________ Day of Week

Medication ____________ Dosage __________

Skipped Medication Yes No

Time(s) medication taken:

AM __________ AM __________
PM __________ PM __________

Time(s) medication wore off: _______ _______

Taken: ☐1 ☐2 On empty stomach
☐1 ☐2 With Food

Kind of food ________________________________

____

Appetite: Poor Average Good

Slept from _______ to ________ Total: ______

Felt rested after waking: Yes No

Side Effects: ________________________________

____

____

____

____

Symptom Details

Rate the following on a scale of 1 to 5:
(1-Poor 2- Meh 3- Decent 4- Good 5-Super)

Mood _____ Focus _____ Memory _____

Energy _____ Motivation _____ Finishing Tasks _____

Patience _____ Impulsivity _____ Restlessness _____

Time Management _____ Emotion Management _____

Other: ______________ _____ ________________ ____

Medication helped today: Yes No Somewhat

Today's Successes: ________________________________

____

____

____

____

Areas for Improvement: __________________________

____

____

____

Rating for This Day
1- Awful / 5- Great

☆☆☆☆☆

Medication Details

Date ______________ ______________ Day of Week

Medication ______________ Dosage ___________

Skipped Medication Yes No

Time(s) medication taken:

AM ___________ AM ___________
PM ___________ PM ___________

Time(s) medication wore off: ________ ________

Taken: ☐1 ☐2 On empty stomach
☐1 ☐2 With Food

Kind of food _______________________________________

____

Appetite: Poor Average Good

Slept from ________ to __________ Total: _______

Felt rested after waking: Yes No

Side Effects: ____

____

____

____

____

Symptom Details

Rate the following on a scale of 1 to 5:
(1-Poor 2- Meh 3- Decent 4- Good 5-Super)

Mood _____ Focus _____ Memory _____

Energy _____ Motivation _____ Finishing Tasks _____

Patience _____ Impulsivity _____ Restlessness _____

Time Management _____ Emotion Management _____

Other: _______________ _____ _________________ ____

Medication helped today: Yes No Somewhat

Today's Successes: ________________________________

____

____

____

____

Areas for Improvement: ____________________________

____

____

____

Rating for This Day
1- Awful / 5- Great

☆☆☆☆☆

Medication Details

Date ____________ ____________ Day of Week

Medication ____________ Dosage __________

Skipped Medication Yes No

Time(s) medication taken:

AM __________ AM __________

PM __________ PM __________

Time(s) medication wore off: ________ ________

Taken: ☐1 ☐2 On empty stomach

☐1 ☐2 With Food

Kind of food __________________________________

____

Appetite: Poor Average Good

Slept from ________ to _________ Total: _______

Felt rested after waking: Yes No

Side Effects: ____________________________________

____

____

____

____

Symptom Details

Rate the following on a scale of 1 to 5:
(1-Poor 2- Meh 3- Decent 4- Good 5-Super)

Mood _____ Focus _____ Memory _____

Energy _____ Motivation _____ Finishing Tasks _____

Patience _____ Impulsivity _____ Restlessness _____

Time Management _____ Emotion Management _____

Other: _______________ _____ _______________ ____

Medication helped today: Yes No Somewhat

Today's Successes: ______________________________

____

____

____

____

Areas for Improvement: ___________________________

____

____

____

Rating for This Day
1- Awful / 5- Great

☆☆☆☆☆

Medication Details

Date ____________ ____________ Day of Week

Medication ____________ Dosage __________

Skipped Medication Yes No

Time(s) medication taken:

AM __________ AM __________
PM __________ PM __________

Time(s) medication wore off: ________ ________

Taken: [1] [2] On empty stomach
[1] [2] With Food

Kind of food ____________________________________

____

Appetite: Poor Average Good

Slept from ________ to _________ Total: _______

Felt rested after waking: Yes No

Side Effects: ____________________________________

____

____

____

____

Symptom Details

Rate the following on a scale of 1 to 5:
(1-Poor 2- Meh 3- Decent 4- Good 5-Super)

Mood _____ Focus _____ Memory _____

Energy _____ Motivation _____ Finishing Tasks _____

Patience _____ Impulsivity _____ Restlessness _____

Time Management _____ Emotion Management _____

Other: _______________ _____ _______________ ____

Medication helped today: Yes No Somewhat

Today's Successes: ______________________________

____

____

____

____

Areas for Improvement: __________________________

____

____

____

Rating for This Day
1- Awful / 5- Great

☆☆☆☆☆

Medication Details

Date ____________ ____________ Day of Week

Medication ____________ Dosage __________

Skipped Medication Yes No

Time(s) medication taken:

AM __________ AM __________
PM __________ PM __________

Time(s) medication wore off: ________ ________

Taken: [1] [2] On empty stomach
[1] [2] With Food

Kind of food ______________________________________

____

Appetite: Poor Average Good

Slept from ________ to _________ Total: _______

Felt rested after waking: Yes No

Side Effects: ______________________________________

____

____

____

____

Symptom Details

Rate the following on a scale of 1 to 5:
(1-Poor 2- Meh 3- Decent 4- Good 5-Super)

Mood _____ Focus _____ Memory _____

Energy _____ Motivation _____ Finishing Tasks _____

Patience _____ Impulsivity _____ Restlessness _____

Time Management _____ Emotion Management _____

Other: ______________ _____ ______________ ____

Medication helped today: Yes No Somewhat

Today's Successes: ______________________________

____

____

____

____

Areas for Improvement: __________________________

____

____

____

Rating for This Day
1- Awful / 5- Great

☆☆☆☆☆

Medication Details

Date ____________ ____________ Day of Week

Medication ____________ Dosage __________

Skipped Medication Yes No

Time(s) medication taken:

AM __________ AM __________
PM __________ PM __________

Time(s) medication wore off: _______ _______

Taken: ☐1 ☐2 On empty stomach
☐1 ☐2 With Food

Kind of food ________________________________

____

Appetite: Poor Average Good

Slept from _______ to ________ Total: ______

Felt rested after waking: Yes No

Side Effects: ________________________________

____

____

____

____

Symptom Details

Rate the following on a scale of 1 to 5:
(1-Poor 2- Meh 3- Decent 4- Good 5-Super)

Mood _____ Focus _____ Memory _____

Energy _____ Motivation _____ Finishing Tasks _____

Patience _____ Impulsivity _____ Restlessness _____

Time Management _____ Emotion Management _____

Other: ______________ _____ ______________ ____

Medication helped today: Yes No Somewhat

Today's Successes: ______________________________

____

____

____

____

Areas for Improvement: __________________________

____

____

____

Rating for This Day
1- Awful / 5- Great

☆☆☆☆☆

Medication Details

Date ______________ ______________ Day of Week

Medication ______________ Dosage ___________

Skipped Medication Yes No

Time(s) medication taken:

AM ___________ AM ___________
PM ___________ PM ___________

Time(s) medication wore off: ________ ________

Taken: [1] [2] On empty stomach
[1] [2] With Food

Kind of food ______________________________________

____

Appetite: Poor Average Good

Slept from ________ to _________ Total: _______

Felt rested after waking: Yes No

Side Effects: ______________________________________

____

____

____

____

Symptom Details

Rate the following on a scale of 1 to 5:
(1-Poor 2- Meh 3- Decent 4- Good 5-Super)

Mood _____ Focus _____ Memory _____

Energy _____ Motivation _____ Finishing Tasks _____

Patience _____ Impulsivity _____ Restlessness _____

Time Management _____ Emotion Management _____

Other: _______________ _____ _______________ ____

Medication helped today: Yes No Somewhat

Today's Successes: ______________________________

____

____

____

____

Areas for Improvement: __________________________

____

____

____

Rating for This Day
1- Awful / 5- Great

Medication Details

Date ____________ ____________ Day of Week

Medication ____________ Dosage __________

Skipped Medication Yes No

Time(s) medication taken:

AM __________ AM __________
PM __________ PM __________

Time(s) medication wore off: _______ _______

Taken: [1] [2] On empty stomach
[1] [2] With Food

Kind of food ____

____

Appetite: Poor Average Good

Slept from _______ to ________ Total: ______

Felt rested after waking: Yes No

Side Effects: ____

____

____

____

____

Symptom Details

Rate the following on a scale of 1 to 5:
(1-Poor 2- Meh 3- Decent 4- Good 5-Super)

Mood _____ Focus _____ Memory _____

Energy _____ Motivation _____ Finishing Tasks _____

Patience _____ Impulsivity _____ Restlessness _____

Time Management _____ Emotion Management _____

Other: ______________ _____ ________________ ____

Medication helped today: Yes No Somewhat

Today's Successes: ________________________________

____

____

____

____

Areas for Improvement: __________________________

____

____

____

Rating for This Day
1- Awful / 5- Great

☆☆☆☆☆

Medication Details

Date ____________ ____________ Day of Week

Medication ____________ Dosage __________

Skipped Medication Yes No

Time(s) medication taken:

AM __________ AM __________
PM __________ PM __________

Time(s) medication wore off: _______ _______

Taken: ☐1 ☐2 On empty stomach
☐1 ☐2 With Food

Kind of food ________________________________

____

Appetite: Poor Average Good

Slept from _______ to _________ Total: ______

Felt rested after waking: Yes No

Side Effects: ________________________________

____

____

____

____

Symptom Details

Rate the following on a scale of 1 to 5:
(1-Poor 2- Meh 3- Decent 4- Good 5-Super)

Mood _____ Focus _____ Memory _____

Energy _____ Motivation _____ Finishing Tasks _____

Patience _____ Impulsivity _____ Restlessness _____

Time Management _____ Emotion Management _____

Other: _______________ _____ _______________ _____

Medication helped today: Yes No Somewhat

Today's Successes: ______________________________

____

____

____

____

Areas for Improvement: ______________________________

____

____

____

Rating for This Day
1- Awful / 5- Great

☆☆☆☆☆

Medication Details

Date ____________ ____________ Day of Week

Medication ____________ Dosage __________

Skipped Medication Yes No

Time(s) medication taken:

AM __________ AM __________
PM __________ PM __________

Time(s) medication wore off: ________ ________

Taken: ☐1 ☐2 On empty stomach
☐1 ☐2 With Food

Kind of food ___________________________________

____

Appetite: Poor Average Good

Slept from ________ to _________ Total: _______

Felt rested after waking: Yes No

Side Effects: ____________________________________

____

____

____

____

Symptom Details

Rate the following on a scale of 1 to 5:
(1-Poor 2- Meh 3- Decent 4- Good 5-Super)

Mood _____ Focus _____ Memory _____

Energy _____ Motivation _____ Finishing Tasks _____

Patience _____ Impulsivity _____ Restlessness _____

Time Management _____ Emotion Management _____

Other: _______________ _____ _________________ ____

Medication helped today: Yes No Somewhat

Today's Successes: ______________________________

____

____

____

____

Areas for Improvement: ________________________

____

____

____

Rating for This Day
1- Awful / 5- Great

☆☆☆☆☆

Medication Details

Date ____________ ____________ Day of Week

Medication ____________ Dosage __________

Skipped Medication Yes No

Time(s) medication taken:

AM __________ AM __________
PM __________ PM __________

Time(s) medication wore off: _______ _______

Taken: ☐1 ☐2 On empty stomach
☐1 ☐2 With Food

Kind of food ________________________________

____

Appetite: Poor Average Good

Slept from _______ to ________ Total: ______

Felt rested after waking: Yes No

Side Effects: ________________________________

____

____

____

____

Symptom Details

Rate the following on a scale of 1 to 5:
(1-Poor 2- Meh 3- Decent 4- Good 5-Super)

Mood _____ Focus _____ Memory _____

Energy _____ Motivation _____ Finishing Tasks _____

Patience _____ Impulsivity _____ Restlessness _____

Time Management _____ Emotion Management _____

Other: ______________ _____ ________________ ____

Medication helped today: Yes No Somewhat

Today's Successes: ________________________________

____

____

____

____

Areas for Improvement: __________________________

____

____

____

Rating for This Day
1- Awful / 5- Great

☆☆☆☆☆

Medication Details

Date ____________ ____________ Day of Week

Medication ____________ Dosage __________

Skipped Medication Yes No

Time(s) medication taken:

AM __________ AM __________
PM __________ PM __________

Time(s) medication wore off: ________ ________

Taken: ☐1 ☐2 On empty stomach
☐1 ☐2 With Food

Kind of food __________________________________

____

Appetite: Poor Average Good

Slept from ________ to _________ Total: ______

Felt rested after waking: Yes No

Side Effects: ____________________________________

____

____

____

____

Symptom Details

Rate the following on a scale of 1 to 5:
(1-Poor 2- Meh 3- Decent 4- Good 5-Super)

Mood _____ Focus _____ Memory _____

Energy _____ Motivation _____ Finishing Tasks _____

Patience _____ Impulsivity _____ Restlessness _____

Time Management _____ Emotion Management _____

Other: _______________ _____ _________________ ____

Medication helped today: Yes No Somewhat

Today's Successes: ______________________________

____

____

____

____

Areas for Improvement: _________________________

____

____

____

Rating for This Day
1- Awful / 5- Great

☆☆☆☆☆

Medication Details

Date ____________ ____________ Day of Week

Medication ____________ Dosage __________

Skipped Medication Yes No

Time(s) medication taken:

AM __________ AM __________
PM __________ PM __________

Time(s) medication wore off: _______ _______

Taken: [1] [2] On empty stomach
[1] [2] With Food

Kind of food ________________________________

____

Appetite: Poor Average Good

Slept from _______ to ________ Total: ______

Felt rested after waking: Yes No

Side Effects: ________________________________

____

____

____

____

Symptom Details

Rate the following on a scale of 1 to 5:
(1-Poor 2- Meh 3- Decent 4- Good 5-Super)

Mood _____ Focus _____ Memory _____

Energy _____ Motivation _____ Finishing Tasks _____

Patience _____ Impulsivity _____ Restlessness _____

Time Management _____ Emotion Management _____

Other: ________________ _____ ________________ ____

Medication helped today: Yes No Somewhat

Today's Successes: ______________________________

____

____

____

____

Areas for Improvement: __________________________

____

____

____

Rating for This Day
1- Awful / 5- Great

☆☆☆☆☆

Medication Details

Date ____________ ____________ Day of Week

Medication ____________ Dosage __________

Skipped Medication Yes No

Time(s) medication taken:

AM __________ AM __________
PM __________ PM __________

Time(s) medication wore off: ________ ________

Taken: 1 2 On empty stomach
1 2 With Food

Kind of food ___________________________________

____

Appetite: Poor Average Good

Slept from ________ to _________ Total: ______

Felt rested after waking: Yes No

Side Effects: ___________________________________

____

____

____

____

Symptom Details

Rate the following on a scale of 1 to 5:
(1-Poor 2- Meh 3- Decent 4- Good 5-Super)

Mood _____ Focus _____ Memory _____

Energy _____ Motivation _____ Finishing Tasks _____

Patience _____ Impulsivity _____ Restlessness _____

Time Management _____ Emotion Management _____

Other: _______________ _____ _______________ ____

Medication helped today: Yes No Somewhat

Today's Successes: ______________________________

____

____

____

____

Areas for Improvement: __________________________

____

____

____

Rating for This Day
1- Awful / 5- Great

☆☆☆☆☆

Medication Details

Date ______________ ______________ Day of Week

Medication ______________ Dosage __________

Skipped Medication Yes No

Time(s) medication taken:

AM ___________ AM ___________
PM ___________ PM ___________

Time(s) medication wore off: ________ ________

Taken: [1] [2] On empty stomach
[1] [2] With Food

Kind of food ______________________________________

____

Appetite: Poor Average Good

Slept from ________ to _________ Total: _______

Felt rested after waking: Yes No

Side Effects: ______________________________________

____

____

____

____

Symptom Details

Rate the following on a scale of 1 to 5:
(1-Poor 2- Meh 3- Decent 4- Good 5-Super)

Mood _____ Focus _____ Memory _____

Energy _____ Motivation _____ Finishing Tasks _____

Patience _____ Impulsivity _____ Restlessness _____

Time Management _____ Emotion Management _____

Other: _______________ _____ _______________ ____

Medication helped today: Yes No Somewhat

Today's Successes: ______________________________

____

____

____

____

Areas for Improvement: ___________________________

____

____

____

Rating for This Day
1- Awful / 5- Great

☆☆☆☆☆

Medication Details

Date ____________ ____________ Day of Week

Medication ____________ Dosage __________

Skipped Medication Yes No

Time(s) medication taken:

AM __________ AM __________
PM __________ PM __________

Time(s) medication wore off: ________ ________

Taken: ☐1 ☐2 On empty stomach
☐1 ☐2 With Food

Kind of food ______________________________________

____

Appetite: Poor Average Good

Slept from ________ to _________ Total: _______

Felt rested after waking: Yes No

Side Effects: ____________________________________

____

____

____

____

Symptom Details

Rate the following on a scale of 1 to 5:
(1-Poor 2- Meh 3- Decent 4- Good 5-Super)

Mood _____ Focus _____ Memory _____

Energy _____ Motivation _____ Finishing Tasks _____

Patience _____ Impulsivity _____ Restlessness _____

Time Management _____ Emotion Management _____

Other: _______________ _____ _________________ ____

Medication helped today: Yes No Somewhat

Today's Successes: __________________________________

____

____

____

____

Areas for Improvement: ____________________________

____

____

____

Rating for This Day
1- Awful / 5- Great

☆☆☆☆☆

Medication Details

Date ____________ ____________ Day of Week

Medication ____________ Dosage __________

Skipped Medication Yes No

Time(s) medication taken:

AM __________ AM __________
PM __________ PM __________

Time(s) medication wore off: ________ ________

Taken: [1] [2] On empty stomach
[1] [2] With Food

Kind of food ____________________________________

____

Appetite: Poor Average Good

Slept from ________ to _________ Total: ______

Felt rested after waking: Yes No

Side Effects: ____________________________________

____

____

____

____

Symptom Details

Rate the following on a scale of 1 to 5:
(1-Poor 2- Meh 3- Decent 4- Good 5-Super)

Mood _____ Focus _____ Memory _____

Energy _____ Motivation _____ Finishing Tasks _____

Patience _____ Impulsivity _____ Restlessness _____

Time Management _____ Emotion Management _____

Other: ______________ _____ ______________ ____

Medication helped today: Yes No Somewhat

Today's Successes: ______________________________

____

____

____

____

Areas for Improvement: __________________________

____

____

____

Rating for This Day
1- Awful / 5- Great

☆☆☆☆☆

Medication Details

Date ____________ ____________ Day of Week

Medication ____________ Dosage __________

Skipped Medication Yes No

Time(s) medication taken:

AM __________ AM __________
PM __________ PM __________

Time(s) medication wore off: ________ ________

Taken: [1] [2] On empty stomach
[1] [2] With Food

Kind of food ______________________________________

____

Appetite: Poor Average Good

Slept from ________ to _________ Total: _______

Felt rested after waking: Yes No

Side Effects: ______________________________________

____

____

____

____

Symptom Details

Rate the following on a scale of 1 to 5:
(1-Poor 2- Meh 3- Decent 4- Good 5-Super)

Mood _____ Focus _____ Memory _____

Energy _____ Motivation _____ Finishing Tasks _____

Patience _____ Impulsivity _____ Restlessness _____

Time Management _____ Emotion Management _____

Other: ______________ _____ ________________ ____

Medication helped today: Yes No Somewhat

Today's Successes: ________________________________

____

____

____

____

Areas for Improvement: __________________________

____

____

____

Rating for This Day
1- Awful / 5- Great

☆☆☆☆☆

Medication Details

Date ____________ ____________ Day of Week

Medication ____________ Dosage __________

Skipped Medication Yes No

Time(s) medication taken:

AM __________ AM __________
PM __________ PM __________

Time(s) medication wore off: _______ _______

Taken: ☐1 ☐2 On empty stomach
☐1 ☐2 With Food

Kind of food ______________________________

____

Appetite: Poor Average Good

Slept from _______ to ________ Total: ______

Felt rested after waking: Yes No

Side Effects: _________________________________

____

____

____

____

Symptom Details

Rate the following on a scale of 1 to 5:
(1-Poor 2- Meh 3- Decent 4- Good 5-Super)

Mood _____ Focus _____ Memory _____

Energy _____ Motivation _____ Finishing Tasks _____

Patience _____ Impulsivity _____ Restlessness _____

Time Management _____ Emotion Management _____

Other: ______________ _____ ________________ ____

Medication helped today: Yes No Somewhat

Today's Successes: ________________________________

____

____

____

____

Areas for Improvement: __________________________

____

____

____

Rating for This Day
1- Awful / 5- Great

☆☆☆☆☆

Medication Details

Date ____________ ____________ Day of Week

Medication ____________ Dosage __________

Skipped Medication Yes No

Time(s) medication taken:

AM __________ AM __________
PM __________ PM __________

Time(s) medication wore off: _______ _______

Taken: [1] [2] On empty stomach
[1] [2] With Food

Kind of food ________________________________

____

Appetite: Poor Average Good

Slept from _______ to ________ Total: ______

Felt rested after waking: Yes No

Side Effects: ________________________________

____

____

____

____

Symptom Details

Rate the following on a scale of 1 to 5:
(1-Poor 2- Meh 3- Decent 4- Good 5-Super)

Mood _____ Focus _____ Memory _____

Energy _____ Motivation _____ Finishing Tasks _____

Patience _____ Impulsivity _____ Restlessness _____

Time Management _____ Emotion Management _____

Other: ______________ _____ ______________ ____

Medication helped today: Yes No Somewhat

Today's Successes: ______________________________

____

____

____

____

Areas for Improvement: __________________________

____

____

____

Rating for This Day
1- Awful / 5- Great

☆☆☆☆☆

Medication Details

Date ______________ ______________ Day of Week

Medication ______________ Dosage ___________

Skipped Medication Yes No

Time(s) medication taken:

AM ___________ AM ___________
PM ___________ PM ___________

Time(s) medication wore off: ________ ________

Taken: [1] [2] On empty stomach
[1] [2] With Food

Kind of food ______________________________________

____

Appetite: Poor Average Good

Slept from ________ to _________ Total: _______

Felt rested after waking: Yes No

Side Effects: ______________________________________

____

____

____

____

Symptom Details

Rate the following on a scale of 1 to 5:
(1-Poor 2- Meh 3- Decent 4- Good 5-Super)

Mood _____ Focus _____ Memory _____

Energy _____ Motivation _____ Finishing Tasks _____

Patience _____ Impulsivity _____ Restlessness _____

Time Management _____ Emotion Management _____

Other: _______________ _____ _________________ ____

Medication helped today: Yes No Somewhat

Today's Successes: ___________________________________

____

____

____

____

Areas for Improvement: ____________________________

____

____

____

Rating for This Day
1- Awful / 5- Great

☆☆☆☆☆

Medication Details

Date ____________ ____________ Day of Week

Medication ____________ Dosage __________

Skipped Medication Yes No

Time(s) medication taken:

AM __________ AM __________
PM __________ PM __________

Time(s) medication wore off: ________ ________

Taken: ☐1 ☐2 On empty stomach
☐1 ☐2 With Food

Kind of food ____________________________________

____

Appetite: Poor Average Good

Slept from ________ to _________ Total: ______

Felt rested after waking: Yes No

Side Effects: ____________________________________

____

____

____

____

Symptom Details

Rate the following on a scale of 1 to 5:
(1-Poor 2- Meh 3- Decent 4- Good 5-Super)

Mood _____ Focus _____ Memory _____

Energy _____ Motivation _____ Finishing Tasks _____

Patience _____ Impulsivity _____ Restlessness _____

Time Management _____ Emotion Management _____

Other: _______________ _____ _________________ ____

Medication helped today: Yes No Somewhat

Today's Successes: ________________________________

____

____

____

____

Areas for Improvement: __________________________

____

____

____

Rating for This Day
1- Awful / 5- Great

☆☆☆☆☆

Medication Details

Date ____________ ____________ Day of Week

Medication ____________ Dosage __________

Skipped Medication Yes No

Time(s) medication taken:

AM __________ AM __________
PM __________ PM __________

Time(s) medication wore off: ________ ________

Taken: [1] [2] On empty stomach
[1] [2] With Food

Kind of food ______________________________________

____

Appetite: Poor Average Good

Slept from ________ to _________ Total: _______

Felt rested after waking: Yes No

Side Effects: ____________________________________

____

____

____

____

Symptom Details

Rate the following on a scale of 1 to 5:
(1-Poor 2- Meh 3- Decent 4- Good 5-Super)

Mood _____ Focus _____ Memory _____

Energy _____ Motivation _____ Finishing Tasks _____

Patience _____ Impulsivity _____ Restlessness _____

Time Management _____ Emotion Management _____

Other: ______________ _____ ________________ ____

Medication helped today: Yes No Somewhat

Today's Successes: ________________________________

____

____

____

____

Areas for Improvement: __________________________

____

____

____

Rating for This Day
1- Awful / 5- Great

☆☆☆☆☆

Medication Details

Date ____________ ____________ Day of Week

Medication ____________ Dosage __________

Skipped Medication Yes No

Time(s) medication taken:

AM __________ AM __________
PM __________ PM __________

Time(s) medication wore off: ________ ________

Taken: [1] [2] On empty stomach
[1] [2] With Food

Kind of food ____________________________________

____

Appetite: Poor Average Good

Slept from ________ to _________ Total: _______

Felt rested after waking: Yes No

Side Effects: ____________________________________

____

____

____

____

Symptom Details

Rate the following on a scale of 1 to 5:
(1-Poor 2- Meh 3- Decent 4- Good 5-Super)

Mood _____ Focus _____ Memory _____

Energy _____ Motivation _____ Finishing Tasks _____

Patience _____ Impulsivity _____ Restlessness _____

Time Management _____ Emotion Management _____

Other: ______________ _____ ________________ ____

Medication helped today: Yes No Somewhat

Today's Successes: ______________________________

____

____

____

____

Areas for Improvement: ___________________________

____

____

____

Rating for This Day
1- Awful / 5- Great

☆☆☆☆☆

Medication Details

Date ____________ ____________ Day of Week

Medication ____________ Dosage __________

Skipped Medication Yes No

Time(s) medication taken:

AM __________ AM __________
PM __________ PM __________

Time(s) medication wore off: ________ ________

Taken: ☐1 ☐2 On empty stomach
☐1 ☐2 With Food

Kind of food ______________________________________

____

Appetite: Poor Average Good

Slept from ________ to _________ Total: _______

Felt rested after waking: Yes No

Side Effects: ____________________________________

____

____

____

____

Symptom Details

Rate the following on a scale of 1 to 5:
(1-Poor 2- Meh 3- Decent 4- Good 5-Super)

Mood _____ Focus _____ Memory _____

Energy _____ Motivation _____ Finishing Tasks _____

Patience _____ Impulsivity _____ Restlessness _____

Time Management _____ Emotion Management _____

Other: _______________ _____ _________________ ____

Medication helped today: Yes No Somewhat

Today's Successes: __________________________________

____

____

____

____

Areas for Improvement: ____________________________

____

____

____

Rating for This Day
1- Awful / 5- Great

☆☆☆☆☆

Medication Details

Date ____________ ____________ Day of Week

Medication ____________ Dosage __________

Skipped Medication Yes No

Time(s) medication taken:

AM __________ AM __________
PM __________ PM __________

Time(s) medication wore off: ________ ________

Taken: [1] [2] On empty stomach
[1] [2] With Food

Kind of food ______________________________________

____

Appetite: Poor Average Good

Slept from ________ to _________ Total: _______

Felt rested after waking: Yes No

Side Effects: ____________________________________

____

____

____

____

Symptom Details

Rate the following on a scale of 1 to 5:
(1-Poor 2- Meh 3- Decent 4- Good 5-Super)

Mood _____ Focus _____ Memory _____

Energy _____ Motivation _____ Finishing Tasks _____

Patience _____ Impulsivity _____ Restlessness _____

Time Management _____ Emotion Management _____

Other: ______________ _____ ________________ ____

Medication helped today: Yes No Somewhat

Today's Successes: ________________________________

____

____

____

____

Areas for Improvement: ___________________________

____

____

____

Rating for This Day
1- Awful / 5- Great

☆☆☆☆☆

Medication Details

Date ____________ ____________ Day of Week

Medication ____________ Dosage __________

Skipped Medication Yes No

Time(s) medication taken:

AM __________ AM __________
PM __________ PM __________

Time(s) medication wore off: _______ _______

Taken: [1] [2] On empty stomach
[1] [2] With Food

Kind of food ________________________________

____

Appetite: Poor Average Good

Slept from _______ to ________ Total: ______

Felt rested after waking: Yes No

Side Effects: ________________________________

____

____

____

____

Symptom Details

Rate the following on a scale of 1 to 5:
(1-Poor 2- Meh 3- Decent 4- Good 5-Super)

Mood _____ Focus _____ Memory _____

Energy _____ Motivation _____ Finishing Tasks _____

Patience _____ Impulsivity _____ Restlessness _____

Time Management _____ Emotion Management _____

Other: ______________ _____ ________________ ____

Medication helped today: Yes No Somewhat

Today's Successes: ______________________________

____

____

____

____

Areas for Improvement: __________________________

____

____

____

Rating for This Day
1- Awful / 5- Great

☆☆☆☆☆

Medication Details

Date ______________ ______________ Day of Week

Medication ______________ Dosage ___________

Skipped Medication Yes No

Time(s) medication taken:

AM ___________ AM ___________
PM ___________ PM ___________

Time(s) medication wore off: ________ ________

Taken: [1] [2] On empty stomach
[1] [2] With Food

Kind of food ______________________________________

____

Appetite: Poor Average Good

Slept from ________ to _________ Total: _______

Felt rested after waking: Yes No

Side Effects: _______________________________________

____

____

____

____

Symptom Details

Rate the following on a scale of 1 to 5:
(1-Poor 2- Meh 3- Decent 4- Good 5-Super)

Mood _____ Focus _____ Memory _____

Energy _____ Motivation _____ Finishing Tasks _____

Patience _____ Impulsivity _____ Restlessness _____

Time Management _____ Emotion Management _____

Other: ______________ _____ ________________ ____

Medication helped today: Yes No Somewhat

Today's Successes: ________________________________

____

____

____

____

Areas for Improvement: __________________________

____

____

____

Rating for This Day
1- Awful / 5- Great

☆☆☆☆☆

Medication Details

Date ____________ ____________ Day of Week

Medication ____________ Dosage __________

Skipped Medication Yes No

Time(s) medication taken:

AM __________ AM __________
PM __________ PM __________

Time(s) medication wore off: _______ _______

Taken: ☐1 ☐2 On empty stomach
☐1 ☐2 With Food

Kind of food ________________________________

____

Appetite: Poor Average Good

Slept from _______ to ________ Total: ______

Felt rested after waking: Yes No

Side Effects: ________________________________

____

____

____

____

Symptom Details

Rate the following on a scale of 1 to 5:
(1-Poor 2- Meh 3- Decent 4- Good 5-Super)

Mood _____ Focus _____ Memory _____

Energy _____ Motivation _____ Finishing Tasks _____

Patience _____ Impulsivity _____ Restlessness _____

Time Management _____ Emotion Management _____

Other: _______________ _____ _______________ ____

Medication helped today: Yes No Somewhat

Today's Successes: _______________________________

____

____

____

____

Areas for Improvement: ___________________________

____

____

____

Rating for This Day
1- Awful / 5- Great

☆☆☆☆☆

Medication Details

Date ____________ ____________ Day of Week

Medication ____________ Dosage __________

Skipped Medication Yes No

Time(s) medication taken:

AM __________ AM __________
PM __________ PM __________

Time(s) medication wore off: _______ _______

Taken: [1] [2] On empty stomach
[1] [2] With Food

Kind of food ________________________________

____

Appetite: Poor Average Good

Slept from _______ to ________ Total: ______

Felt rested after waking: Yes No

Side Effects: ________________________________

____

____

____

____

Symptom Details

Rate the following on a scale of 1 to 5:
(1-Poor 2- Meh 3- Decent 4- Good 5-Super)

Mood _____ Focus _____ Memory _____

Energy _____ Motivation _____ Finishing Tasks _____

Patience _____ Impulsivity _____ Restlessness _____

Time Management _____ Emotion Management _____

Other: _______________ _____ _______________ ____

Medication helped today: Yes No Somewhat

Today's Successes: ______________________________

____

____

____

____

Areas for Improvement: ________________________

____

____

____

Rating for This Day
1- Awful / 5- Great

☆☆☆☆☆

Medication Details

Date ______________ ______________ Day of Week

Medication ______________ Dosage ___________

Skipped Medication Yes No

Time(s) medication taken:

AM ___________ AM ___________
PM ___________ PM ___________

Time(s) medication wore off: _________ _________

Taken: [1] [2] On empty stomach
[1] [2] With Food

Kind of food ____

____

Appetite: Poor Average Good

Slept from _________ to __________ Total: _______

Felt rested after waking: Yes No

Side Effects: ____

____

____

____

____

Symptom Details

Rate the following on a scale of 1 to 5:
(1-Poor 2- Meh 3- Decent 4- Good 5-Super)

Mood _____ Focus _____ Memory _____

Energy _____ Motivation _____ Finishing Tasks _____

Patience _____ Impulsivity _____ Restlessness _____

Time Management _____ Emotion Management _____

Other: ______________ _____ ______________ ____

Medication helped today: Yes No Somewhat

Today's Successes: ______________________________

____

____

____

____

Areas for Improvement: __________________________

____

____

____

Rating for This Day
1- Awful / 5- Great

☆☆☆☆☆

Medication Details

Date ____________ ____________ Day of Week

Medication ____________ Dosage __________

Skipped Medication Yes No

Time(s) medication taken:

AM __________ AM __________
PM __________ PM __________

Time(s) medication wore off: _______ _______

Taken: [1] [2] On empty stomach
[1] [2] With Food

Kind of food ________________________________

____

Appetite: Poor Average Good

Slept from _______ to ________ Total: ______

Felt rested after waking: Yes No

Side Effects: ________________________________

____

____

____

____

Symptom Details

Rate the following on a scale of 1 to 5:
(1-Poor 2- Meh 3- Decent 4- Good 5-Super)

Mood _____ Focus _____ Memory _____

Energy _____ Motivation _____ Finishing Tasks _____

Patience _____ Impulsivity _____ Restlessness _____

Time Management _____ Emotion Management _____

Other: _______________ _____ _______________ ____

Medication helped today: Yes No Somewhat

Today's Successes: ______________________________

____

____

____

____

Areas for Improvement: __________________________

____

____

____

Rating for This Day
1- Awful / 5- Great

☆☆☆☆☆

Medication Details

Date ____________ ____________ Day of Week

Medication ____________ Dosage __________

Skipped Medication Yes No

Time(s) medication taken:

AM __________ AM __________
PM __________ PM __________

Time(s) medication wore off: ________ ________

Taken: [1] [2] On empty stomach
[1] [2] With Food

Kind of food ________________________________

____

Appetite: Poor Average Good

Slept from ________ to ________ Total: ______

Felt rested after waking: Yes No

Side Effects: ________________________________

____

____

____

____

Symptom Details

Rate the following on a scale of 1 to 5:
(1-Poor 2- Meh 3- Decent 4- Good 5-Super)

Mood _____ Focus _____ Memory _____

Energy _____ Motivation _____ Finishing Tasks _____

Patience _____ Impulsivity _____ Restlessness _____

Time Management _____ Emotion Management _____

Other: _______________ _____ _________________ ____

Medication helped today: Yes No Somewhat

Today's Successes: _________________________________

____

____

____

____

Areas for Improvement: ___________________________

____

____

____

Rating for This Day
1- Awful / 5- Great

☆☆☆☆☆

Medication Details

Date ____________ ____________ Day of Week

Medication ____________ Dosage __________

Skipped Medication Yes No

Time(s) medication taken:

AM __________ AM __________
PM __________ PM __________

Time(s) medication wore off: ________ ________

Taken: [1] [2] On empty stomach
[1] [2] With Food

Kind of food ________________________________

____

Appetite: Poor Average Good

Slept from ________ to _________ Total: _______

Felt rested after waking: Yes No

Side Effects: ________________________________

____

____

____

____

Symptom Details

Rate the following on a scale of 1 to 5:
(1-Poor 2- Meh 3- Decent 4- Good 5-Super)

Mood _____ Focus _____ Memory _____

Energy _____ Motivation _____ Finishing Tasks _____

Patience _____ Impulsivity _____ Restlessness _____

Time Management _____ Emotion Management _____

Other: _______________ _____ _______________ ____

Medication helped today: Yes No Somewhat

Today's Successes: ______________________________

____

____

____

____

Areas for Improvement: __________________________

____

____

____

Rating for This Day
1- Awful / 5- Great

☆☆☆☆☆

Medication Details

Date ____________ ____________ Day of Week

Medication ____________ Dosage __________

Skipped Medication Yes No

Time(s) medication taken:

AM __________ AM __________
PM __________ PM __________

Time(s) medication wore off: ________ ________

Taken: ☐1 ☐2 On empty stomach
☐1 ☐2 With Food

Kind of food ________________________________

____

Appetite: Poor Average Good

Slept from ________ to _________ Total: _______

Felt rested after waking: Yes No

Side Effects: ________________________________

____

____

____

____

Symptom Details

Rate the following on a scale of 1 to 5:
(1-Poor 2- Meh 3- Decent 4- Good 5-Super)

Mood _____ Focus _____ Memory _____

Energy _____ Motivation _____ Finishing Tasks _____

Patience _____ Impulsivity _____ Restlessness _____

Time Management _____ Emotion Management _____

Other: _______________ _____ _________________ ____

Medication helped today: Yes No Somewhat

Today's Successes: ________________________________

____

____

____

____

Areas for Improvement: __________________________

____

____

____

Rating for This Day
1- Awful / 5- Great

☆☆☆☆☆

Medication Details

Date ____________ ____________ Day of Week

Medication ____________ Dosage __________

Skipped Medication Yes No

Time(s) medication taken:

AM __________ AM __________
PM __________ PM __________

Time(s) medication wore off: ________ ________

Taken: [1] [2] On empty stomach
[1] [2] With Food

Kind of food ______________________________

____

Appetite: Poor Average Good

Slept from ________ to ________ Total: ______

Felt rested after waking: Yes No

Side Effects: ______________________________

____

____

____

____

Symptom Details

Rate the following on a scale of 1 to 5:
(1-Poor 2- Meh 3- Decent 4- Good 5-Super)

Mood _____ Focus _____ Memory _____

Energy _____ Motivation _____ Finishing Tasks _____

Patience _____ Impulsivity _____ Restlessness _____

Time Management _____ Emotion Management _____

Other: ______________ _____ ______________ _____

Medication helped today: Yes No Somewhat

Today's Successes: ______________________________

____

____

____

____

Areas for Improvement: ______________________

____

____

____

Rating for This Day
1- Awful / 5- Great

☆☆☆☆☆

Medication Details

Date ____________ ____________ Day of Week

Medication ____________ Dosage __________

Skipped Medication Yes No

Time(s) medication taken:

AM __________ AM __________
PM __________ PM __________

Time(s) medication wore off: ________ ________

Taken: [1] [2] On empty stomach
[1] [2] With Food

Kind of food ________________________________

____

Appetite: Poor Average Good

Slept from ________ to _________ Total: _______

Felt rested after waking: Yes No

Side Effects: ________________________________

____

____

____

____

Symptom Details

Rate the following on a scale of 1 to 5:
(1-Poor 2- Meh 3- Decent 4- Good 5-Super)

Mood _____ Focus _____ Memory _____

Energy _____ Motivation _____ Finishing Tasks _____

Patience _____ Impulsivity _____ Restlessness _____

Time Management _____ Emotion Management _____

Other: ______________ _____ ______________ ____

Medication helped today: Yes No Somewhat

Today's Successes: ______________________________

____

____

____

____

Areas for Improvement: __________________________

____

____

____

Rating for This Day
1- Awful / 5- Great

☆☆☆☆☆

Medication Details

Date ______________ ______________ Day of Week

Medication ______________ Dosage ___________

Skipped Medication Yes No

Time(s) medication taken:

AM ___________ AM ___________
PM ___________ PM ___________

Time(s) medication wore off: ________ ________

Taken: [1] [2] On empty stomach
[1] [2] With Food

Kind of food ______________________________________

____

Appetite: Poor Average Good

Slept from ________ to __________ Total: _______

Felt rested after waking: Yes No

Side Effects: ______________________________________

____

____

____

____

Symptom Details

Rate the following on a scale of 1 to 5:
(1-Poor 2- Meh 3- Decent 4- Good 5-Super)

Mood _____ Focus _____ Memory _____

Energy _____ Motivation _____ Finishing Tasks _____

Patience _____ Impulsivity _____ Restlessness _____

Time Management _____ Emotion Management _____

Other: ______________ _____ ________________ ____

Medication helped today: Yes No Somewhat

Today's Successes: ________________________________

____

____

____

____

Areas for Improvement: __________________________

____

____

____

Rating for This Day
1- Awful / 5- Great

☆☆☆☆☆

Medication Details

Date ____________ ____________ Day of Week

Medication ____________ Dosage __________

Skipped Medication Yes No

Time(s) medication taken:

AM __________ AM __________
PM __________ PM __________

Time(s) medication wore off: ________ ________

Taken: ☐1 ☐2 On empty stomach
☐1 ☐2 With Food

Kind of food ________________________________

____

Appetite: Poor Average Good

Slept from ________ to _________ Total: _______

Felt rested after waking: Yes No

Side Effects: ________________________________

____

____

____

____

Symptom Details

Rate the following on a scale of 1 to 5:
(1-Poor 2- Meh 3- Decent 4- Good 5-Super)

Mood _____ Focus _____ Memory _____

Energy _____ Motivation _____ Finishing Tasks _____

Patience _____ Impulsivity _____ Restlessness _____

Time Management _____ Emotion Management _____

Other: _______________ _____ _______________ ____

Medication helped today: Yes No Somewhat

Today's Successes: ______________________________

____

____

____

____

Areas for Improvement: __________________________

____

____

____

Rating for This Day
1- Awful / 5- Great

☆☆☆☆☆

Medication Details

Date ____________ ____________ Day of Week

Medication ____________ Dosage __________

Skipped Medication Yes No

Time(s) medication taken:

AM __________ AM __________
PM __________ PM __________

Time(s) medication wore off: ________ ________

Taken: ☐1 ☐2 On empty stomach
☐1 ☐2 With Food

Kind of food ______________________________

____

Appetite: Poor Average Good

Slept from ________ to _________ Total: _______

Felt rested after waking: Yes No

Side Effects: ______________________________

____

____

____

____

Symptom Details

Rate the following on a scale of 1 to 5:
(1-Poor 2- Meh 3- Decent 4- Good 5-Super)

Mood _____ Focus _____ Memory _____

Energy _____ Motivation _____ Finishing Tasks _____

Patience _____ Impulsivity _____ Restlessness _____

Time Management _____ Emotion Management _____

Other: ______________ _____ ________________ ____

Medication helped today: Yes No Somewhat

Today's Successes: ______________________________

____

____

____

____

Areas for Improvement: _________________________

____

____

____

Rating for This Day
1- Awful / 5- Great

☆☆☆☆☆

Medication Details

Date ____________ ____________ Day of Week

Medication ____________ Dosage __________

Skipped Medication Yes No

Time(s) medication taken:

AM __________ AM __________
PM __________ PM __________

Time(s) medication wore off: ________ ________

Taken: [1] [2] On empty stomach
[1] [2] With Food

Kind of food __________________________________

____

Appetite: Poor Average Good

Slept from ________ to _________ Total: _______

Felt rested after waking: Yes No

Side Effects: ___________________________________

____

____

____

____

Symptom Details

Rate the following on a scale of 1 to 5:
(1-Poor 2- Meh 3- Decent 4- Good 5-Super)

Mood _____ Focus _____ Memory _____

Energy _____ Motivation _____ Finishing Tasks _____

Patience _____ Impulsivity _____ Restlessness _____

Time Management _____ Emotion Management _____

Other: _______________ _____ _______________ ____

Medication helped today: Yes No Somewhat

Today's Successes: ______________________________

____

____

____

____

Areas for Improvement: __________________________

____

____

____

Rating for This Day
1- Awful / 5- Great

☆☆☆☆☆

Medication Details

Date ______________ ______________ Day of Week

Medication ______________ Dosage ___________

Skipped Medication Yes No

Time(s) medication taken:

AM ___________ AM ___________
PM ___________ PM ___________

Time(s) medication wore off: ________ ________

Taken: ☐1 ☐2 On empty stomach
☐1 ☐2 With Food

Kind of food ____

____

Appetite: Poor Average Good

Slept from ________ to __________ Total: _______

Felt rested after waking: Yes No

Side Effects: ____

____

____

____

____

Symptom Details

Rate the following on a scale of 1 to 5:
(1-Poor 2- Meh 3- Decent 4- Good 5-Super)

Mood _____ Focus _____ Memory _____

Energy _____ Motivation _____ Finishing Tasks _____

Patience _____ Impulsivity _____ Restlessness _____

Time Management _____ Emotion Management _____

Other: ______________ _____ ______________ ____

Medication helped today: Yes No Somewhat

Today's Successes: ______________________________

____

____

____

____

Areas for Improvement: __________________________

____

____

____

Rating for This Day
1- Awful / 5- Great

☆☆☆☆☆

Medication Details

Date ______________ ______________ Day of Week

Medication ______________ Dosage ___________

Skipped Medication Yes No

Time(s) medication taken:

AM ___________ AM ___________
PM ___________ PM ___________

Time(s) medication wore off: ________ ________

Taken: ☐1 ☐2 On empty stomach
☐1 ☐2 With Food

Kind of food ______________________________________

____

Appetite: Poor Average Good

Slept from ________ to __________ Total: _______

Felt rested after waking: Yes No

Side Effects: ______________________________________

____

____

____

____

Symptom Details

Rate the following on a scale of 1 to 5:
(1-Poor 2- Meh 3- Decent 4- Good 5-Super)

Mood _____ Focus _____ Memory _____

Energy _____ Motivation _____ Finishing Tasks _____

Patience _____ Impulsivity _____ Restlessness _____

Time Management _____ Emotion Management _____

Other: _______________ _____ _________________ ____

Medication helped today: Yes No Somewhat

Today's Successes: ______________________________

____

____

____

____

Areas for Improvement: _________________________

____

____

____

Rating for This Day
1- Awful / 5- Great

☆☆☆☆☆

Medication Details

Date ____________ ____________ Day of Week

Medication ____________ Dosage __________

Skipped Medication Yes No

Time(s) medication taken:

AM __________ AM __________
PM __________ PM __________

Time(s) medication wore off: ________ ________

Taken: ☐1 ☐2 On empty stomach
☐1 ☐2 With Food

Kind of food __________________________________

____

Appetite: Poor Average Good

Slept from ________ to _________ Total: _______

Felt rested after waking: Yes No

Side Effects: ___________________________________

____

____

____

____

Symptom Details

Rate the following on a scale of 1 to 5:
(1-Poor 2- Meh 3- Decent 4- Good 5-Super)

Mood _____ Focus _____ Memory _____

Energy _____ Motivation _____ Finishing Tasks _____

Patience _____ Impulsivity _____ Restlessness _____

Time Management _____ Emotion Management _____

Other: ________________ _____ ________________ ____

Medication helped today: Yes No Somewhat

Today's Successes: ____________________________________

____

____

____

____

Areas for Improvement: ______________________________

____

____

____

Rating for This Day
1- Awful / 5- Great

☆☆☆☆☆

Medication Details

Date ______________ ______________ Day of Week

Medication ______________ Dosage ___________

Skipped Medication Yes No

Time(s) medication taken:

AM ___________ AM ___________
PM ___________ PM ___________

Time(s) medication wore off: ________ ________

Taken: [1] [2] On empty stomach
[1] [2] With Food

Kind of food ______________________________________
____

Appetite: Poor Average Good

Slept from ________ to _________ Total: _______

Felt rested after waking: Yes No

Side Effects: ______________________________________
____
____
____
____

Symptom Details

Rate the following on a scale of 1 to 5:
(1-Poor 2- Meh 3- Decent 4- Good 5-Super)

Mood _____ Focus _____ Memory _____

Energy _____ Motivation _____ Finishing Tasks _____

Patience _____ Impulsivity _____ Restlessness _____

Time Management _____ Emotion Management _____

Other: ______________ _____ ________________ ____

Medication helped today: Yes No Somewhat

Today's Successes: ________________________________

____

____

____

____

Areas for Improvement: __________________________

____

____

____

Rating for This Day
1- Awful / 5- Great

☆☆☆☆☆

Medication Details

Date ____________ ____________ Day of Week

Medication ____________ Dosage __________

Skipped Medication Yes No

Time(s) medication taken:

AM __________ AM __________
PM __________ PM __________

Time(s) medication wore off: ________ ________

Taken: ☐1 ☐2 On empty stomach
☐1 ☐2 With Food

Kind of food ________________________________

____

Appetite: Poor Average Good

Slept from ________ to _________ Total: _______

Felt rested after waking: Yes No

Side Effects: ________________________________

____

____

____

____

Symptom Details

Rate the following on a scale of 1 to 5:
(1-Poor 2- Meh 3- Decent 4- Good 5-Super)

Mood _____ Focus _____ Memory _____

Energy _____ Motivation _____ Finishing Tasks _____

Patience _____ Impulsivity _____ Restlessness _____

Time Management _____ Emotion Management _____

Other: ______________ _____ ______________ ____

Medication helped today: Yes No Somewhat

Today's Successes: ______________________________

____

____

____

____

Areas for Improvement: ________________________

____

____

____

Rating for This Day
1- Awful / 5- Great

☆☆☆☆☆

Medication Details

Date ___________ ___________ Day of Week

Medication ___________ Dosage _________

Skipped Medication Yes No

Time(s) medication taken:

AM _________ AM _________
PM _________ PM _________

Time(s) medication wore off: _______ _______

Taken: [1] [2] On empty stomach
[1] [2] With Food

Kind of food _______________________________

____

Appetite: Poor Average Good

Slept from _______ to ________ Total: ______

Felt rested after waking: Yes No

Side Effects: _______________________________

____

____

____

____

Symptom Details

Rate the following on a scale of 1 to 5:
(1-Poor 2- Meh 3- Decent 4- Good 5-Super)

Mood _____ Focus _____ Memory _____

Energy _____ Motivation _____ Finishing Tasks _____

Patience _____ Impulsivity _____ Restlessness _____

Time Management _____ Emotion Management _____

Other: ______________ _____ ________________ ____

Medication helped today: Yes No Somewhat

Today's Successes: ________________________________

____

____

____

____

Areas for Improvement: __________________________

____

____

____

Rating for This Day
1- Awful / 5- Great

Medication Details

Date ____________ ____________ Day of Week

Medication ____________ Dosage __________

Skipped Medication Yes No

Time(s) medication taken:

AM __________ AM __________
PM __________ PM __________

Time(s) medication wore off: ________ ________

Taken: [1] [2] On empty stomach
[1] [2] With Food

Kind of food ______________________________

____

Appetite: Poor Average Good

Slept from ________ to _________ Total: ______

Felt rested after waking: Yes No

Side Effects: ______________________________

____

____

____

____

Symptom Details

Rate the following on a scale of 1 to 5:
(1-Poor 2- Meh 3- Decent 4- Good 5-Super)

Mood _____ Focus _____ Memory _____

Energy _____ Motivation _____ Finishing Tasks _____

Patience _____ Impulsivity _____ Restlessness _____

Time Management _____ Emotion Management _____

Other: _______________ _____ _______________ ____

Medication helped today: Yes No Somewhat

Today's Successes: ____________________________________

____

____

____

____

Areas for Improvement: ______________________________

____

____

____

Rating for This Day
1- Awful / 5- Great

☆☆☆☆☆

Medication Details

Date ____________ ____________ Day of Week

Medication ____________ Dosage __________

Skipped Medication Yes No

Time(s) medication taken:

AM __________ AM __________
PM __________ PM __________

Time(s) medication wore off: ________ ________

Taken: [1] [2] On empty stomach
[1] [2] With Food

Kind of food ________________________________

____

Appetite: Poor Average Good

Slept from ________ to _________ Total: _______

Felt rested after waking: Yes No

Side Effects: ________________________________

____

____

____

____

Symptom Details

Rate the following on a scale of 1 to 5:
(1-Poor 2- Meh 3- Decent 4- Good 5-Super)

Mood _____ Focus _____ Memory _____

Energy _____ Motivation _____ Finishing Tasks _____

Patience _____ Impulsivity _____ Restlessness _____

Time Management _____ Emotion Management _____

Other: ______________ _____ ________________ ____

Medication helped today: Yes No Somewhat

Today's Successes: ________________________________

____

____

____

____

Areas for Improvement: __________________________

____

____

____

Rating for This Day
1- Awful / 5- Great

☆☆☆☆☆

Medication Details

Date ____________ ____________ Day of Week

Medication ____________ Dosage __________

Skipped Medication Yes No

Time(s) medication taken:

AM __________ AM __________
PM __________ PM __________

Time(s) medication wore off: ________ ________

Taken: [1] [2] On empty stomach
[1] [2] With Food

Kind of food ______________________________________

____

Appetite: Poor Average Good

Slept from ________ to _________ Total: _______

Felt rested after waking: Yes No

Side Effects: ____________________________________

____

____

____

____

Symptom Details

Rate the following on a scale of 1 to 5:
(1-Poor 2- Meh 3- Decent 4- Good 5-Super)

Mood _____ Focus _____ Memory _____

Energy _____ Motivation _____ Finishing Tasks _____

Patience _____ Impulsivity _____ Restlessness _____

Time Management _____ Emotion Management _____

Other: ______________ _____ ______________ ____

Medication helped today: Yes No Somewhat

Today's Successes: ______________________________

____

____

____

____

Areas for Improvement: __________________________

____

____

____

Rating for This Day
1- Awful / 5- Great

☆☆☆☆☆

Medication Details

Date ____________ ____________ Day of Week

Medication ____________ Dosage __________

Skipped Medication Yes No

Time(s) medication taken:

AM __________ AM __________
PM __________ PM __________

Time(s) medication wore off: ________ ________

Taken: ☐1 ☐2 On empty stomach
☐1 ☐2 With Food

Kind of food ________________________________

____

Appetite: Poor Average Good

Slept from ________ to _________ Total: ______

Felt rested after waking: Yes No

Side Effects: ________________________________

____

____

____

____

Symptom Details

Rate the following on a scale of 1 to 5:
(1-Poor 2- Meh 3- Decent 4- Good 5-Super)

Mood _____ Focus _____ Memory _____

Energy _____ Motivation _____ Finishing Tasks _____

Patience _____ Impulsivity _____ Restlessness _____

Time Management _____ Emotion Management _____

Other: ______________ _____ ______________ ____

Medication helped today: Yes No Somewhat

Today's Successes: ______________________________

____

____

____

____

Areas for Improvement: __________________________

____

____

____

Rating for This Day
1- Awful / 5- Great

☆☆☆☆☆

Medication Details

Date ____________ ____________ Day of Week

Medication ____________ Dosage __________

Skipped Medication Yes No

Time(s) medication taken:

AM __________ AM __________
PM __________ PM __________

Time(s) medication wore off: ________ ________

Taken: [1] [2] On empty stomach
[1] [2] With Food

Kind of food ______________________________

____

Appetite: Poor Average Good

Slept from ________ to _________ Total: ______

Felt rested after waking: Yes No

Side Effects: ______________________________

____

____

____

____

Symptom Details

Rate the following on a scale of 1 to 5:
(1-Poor 2- Meh 3- Decent 4- Good 5-Super)

Mood _____ Focus _____ Memory _____

Energy _____ Motivation _____ Finishing Tasks _____

Patience _____ Impulsivity _____ Restlessness _____

Time Management _____ Emotion Management _____

Other: _______________ _____ _________________ ____

Medication helped today: Yes No Somewhat

Today's Successes: ________________________________

____

____

____

____

Areas for Improvement: __________________________

____

____

____

Rating for This Day
1- Awful / 5- Great

☆☆☆☆☆

Medication Details

Date ____________ ____________ Day of Week

Medication ____________ Dosage __________

Skipped Medication Yes No

Time(s) medication taken:

AM __________ AM __________
PM __________ PM __________

Time(s) medication wore off: ________ ________

Taken: ☐1 ☐2 On empty stomach
☐1 ☐2 With Food

Kind of food ______________________________

____

Appetite: Poor Average Good

Slept from ________ to _________ Total: _______

Felt rested after waking: Yes No

Side Effects: ______________________________

____

____

____

____

Symptom Details

Rate the following on a scale of 1 to 5:
(1-Poor 2- Meh 3- Decent 4- Good 5-Super)

Mood _____ Focus _____ Memory _____

Energy _____ Motivation _____ Finishing Tasks _____

Patience _____ Impulsivity _____ Restlessness _____

Time Management _____ Emotion Management _____

Other: _______________ _____ _________________ ____

Medication helped today: Yes No Somewhat

Today's Successes: __________________________________

____

____

____

____

Areas for Improvement: ____________________________

____

____

____

Rating for This Day
1- Awful / 5- Great

☆☆☆☆☆

Medication Details

Date ____________ ____________ Day of Week

Medication ____________ Dosage __________

Skipped Medication Yes No

Time(s) medication taken:

AM __________ AM __________
PM __________ PM __________

Time(s) medication wore off: ________ ________

Taken: [1] [2] On empty stomach
[1] [2] With Food

Kind of food ______________________________________

____

Appetite: Poor Average Good

Slept from ________ to _________ Total: ______

Felt rested after waking: Yes No

Side Effects: ____________________________________

____

____

____

____

Symptom Details

Rate the following on a scale of 1 to 5:
(1-Poor 2- Meh 3- Decent 4- Good 5-Super)

Mood _____ Focus _____ Memory _____

Energy _____ Motivation _____ Finishing Tasks _____

Patience _____ Impulsivity _____ Restlessness _____

Time Management _____ Emotion Management _____

Other: _______________ _____ _______________ ____

Medication helped today: Yes No Somewhat

Today's Successes: ________________________________

____

____

____

____

Areas for Improvement: ____________________________

____

____

____

Rating for This Day
1- Awful / 5- Great

☆☆☆☆☆

Medication Details

Date ____________ ____________ Day of Week

Medication ____________ Dosage __________

Skipped Medication Yes No

Time(s) medication taken:

AM __________ AM __________
PM __________ PM __________

Time(s) medication wore off: ________ ________

Taken: ☐1 ☐2 On empty stomach
☐1 ☐2 With Food

Kind of food ____________________________________

____

Appetite: Poor Average Good

Slept from ________ to _________ Total: _______

Felt rested after waking: Yes No

Side Effects: ____________________________________

____

____

____

____

Symptom Details

Rate the following on a scale of 1 to 5:
(1-Poor 2- Meh 3- Decent 4- Good 5-Super)

Mood _____ Focus _____ Memory _____

Energy _____ Motivation _____ Finishing Tasks _____

Patience _____ Impulsivity _____ Restlessness _____

Time Management _____ Emotion Management _____

Other: _______________ _____ _________________ ____

Medication helped today: Yes No Somewhat

Today's Successes: ____________________________________

____

____

____

____

Areas for Improvement: ______________________________

____

____

____

Rating for This Day
1- Awful / 5- Great

Medication Details

Date ______________ ______________ Day of Week

Medication ______________ Dosage ___________

Skipped Medication Yes No

Time(s) medication taken:

AM ___________ AM ___________
PM ___________ PM ___________

Time(s) medication wore off: ________ ________

Taken: ☐1 ☐2 On empty stomach
☐1 ☐2 With Food

Kind of food _______________________________________

____

Appetite: Poor Average Good

Slept from ________ to __________ Total: _______

Felt rested after waking: Yes No

Side Effects: _______________________________________

____

____

____

____

Symptom Details

Rate the following on a scale of 1 to 5:
(1-Poor 2- Meh 3- Decent 4- Good 5-Super)

Mood _____ Focus _____ Memory _____

Energy _____ Motivation _____ Finishing Tasks _____

Patience _____ Impulsivity _____ Restlessness _____

Time Management _____ Emotion Management _____

Other: ______________ _____ ________________ ____

Medication helped today: Yes No Somewhat

Today's Successes: ________________________________

____

____

____

____

Areas for Improvement: ____________________________

____

____

____

Rating for This Day
1- Awful / 5- Great

Medication Details

Date ____________ ____________ Day of Week

Medication ____________ Dosage __________

Skipped Medication Yes No

Time(s) medication taken:

AM __________ AM __________
PM __________ PM __________

Time(s) medication wore off: ________ ________

Taken: [1] [2] On empty stomach
[1] [2] With Food

Kind of food ________________________________

____

Appetite: Poor Average Good

Slept from ________ to _________ Total: _______

Felt rested after waking: Yes No

Side Effects: ________________________________

____

____

____

____

Symptom Details

Rate the following on a scale of 1 to 5:
(1-Poor 2- Meh 3- Decent 4- Good 5-Super)

Mood _____ Focus _____ Memory _____

Energy _____ Motivation _____ Finishing Tasks _____

Patience _____ Impulsivity _____ Restlessness _____

Time Management _____ Emotion Management _____

Other: _______________ _____ _________________ ____

Medication helped today: Yes No Somewhat

Today's Successes: ________________________________

____

____

____

____

Areas for Improvement: __________________________

____

____

____

Rating for This Day
1- Awful / 5- Great

☆☆☆☆☆

Medication Details

Date ____________ ____________ Day of Week

Medication ____________ Dosage __________

Skipped Medication Yes No

Time(s) medication taken:

AM __________ AM __________
PM __________ PM __________

Time(s) medication wore off: ________ ________

Taken: ☐1 ☐2 On empty stomach
☐1 ☐2 With Food

Kind of food __________________________________

____

Appetite: Poor Average Good

Slept from ________ to _________ Total: _______

Felt rested after waking: Yes No

Side Effects: ____________________________________

____

____

____

____

Symptom Details

Rate the following on a scale of 1 to 5:
(1-Poor 2- Meh 3- Decent 4- Good 5-Super)

Mood _____ Focus _____ Memory _____

Energy _____ Motivation _____ Finishing Tasks _____

Patience _____ Impulsivity _____ Restlessness _____

Time Management _____ Emotion Management _____

Other: _______________ _____ _________________ ____

Medication helped today: Yes No Somewhat

Today's Successes: ___________________________________

____

____

____

____

Areas for Improvement: _____________________________

____

____

____

Rating for This Day
1- Awful / 5- Great

☆☆☆☆☆

Medication Details

Date ____________ ____________ Day of Week

Medication ____________ Dosage __________

Skipped Medication Yes No

Time(s) medication taken:

AM __________ AM __________
PM __________ PM __________

Time(s) medication wore off: ________ ________

Taken: ☐1 ☐2 On empty stomach
☐1 ☐2 With Food

Kind of food __________________________________

____

Appetite: Poor Average Good

Slept from ________ to _________ Total: _______

Felt rested after waking: Yes No

Side Effects: ___________________________________

____

____

____

____

Symptom Details

Rate the following on a scale of 1 to 5:
(1-Poor 2- Meh 3- Decent 4- Good 5-Super)

Mood _____ Focus _____ Memory _____

Energy _____ Motivation _____ Finishing Tasks _____

Patience _____ Impulsivity _____ Restlessness _____

Time Management _____ Emotion Management _____

Other: ______________ _____ ________________ ____

Medication helped today: Yes No Somewhat

Today's Successes: ________________________________

____

____

____

____

Areas for Improvement: __________________________

____

____

____

Rating for This Day
1- Awful / 5- Great

☆☆☆☆☆

Medication Details

Date ____________ ____________ Day of Week

Medication ____________ Dosage __________

Skipped Medication Yes No

Time(s) medication taken:

AM __________ AM __________
PM __________ PM __________

Time(s) medication wore off: _______ _______

Taken: [1] [2] On empty stomach
[1] [2] With Food

Kind of food ________________________________

____

Appetite: Poor Average Good

Slept from _______ to ________ Total: ______

Felt rested after waking: Yes No

Side Effects: ________________________________

____

____

____

____

Symptom Details

Rate the following on a scale of 1 to 5:
(1-Poor 2- Meh 3- Decent 4- Good 5-Super)

Mood _____ Focus _____ Memory _____

Energy _____ Motivation _____ Finishing Tasks _____

Patience _____ Impulsivity _____ Restlessness _____

Time Management _____ Emotion Management _____

Other: _______________ _____ _________________ ____

Medication helped today: Yes No Somewhat

Today's Successes: ___________________________________

____

____

____

____

Areas for Improvement: ____________________________

____

____

____

Rating for This Day
1- Awful / 5- Great

Medication Details

Date ____________ ____________ Day of Week

Medication ____________ Dosage __________

Skipped Medication Yes No

Time(s) medication taken:

AM __________ AM __________
PM __________ PM __________

Time(s) medication wore off: ________ ________

Taken: [1] [2] On empty stomach
[1] [2] With Food

Kind of food ____________________________________

____

Appetite: Poor Average Good

Slept from ________ to _________ Total: ______

Felt rested after waking: Yes No

Side Effects: ____________________________________

____

____

____

____

Symptom Details

Rate the following on a scale of 1 to 5:
(1-Poor 2- Meh 3- Decent 4- Good 5-Super)

Mood _____ Focus _____ Memory _____

Energy _____ Motivation _____ Finishing Tasks _____

Patience _____ Impulsivity _____ Restlessness _____

Time Management _____ Emotion Management _____

Other: ______________ _____ ________________ ____

Medication helped today: Yes No Somewhat

Today's Successes: ________________________________

____

____

____

____

Areas for Improvement: __________________________

____

____

____

Rating for This Day
1- Awful / 5- Great

☆☆☆☆☆

Medication Details

Date ____________ ____________ Day of Week

Medication ____________ Dosage __________

Skipped Medication Yes No

Time(s) medication taken:

AM __________ AM __________
PM __________ PM __________

Time(s) medication wore off: _______ _______

Taken: [1] [2] On empty stomach
[1] [2] With Food

Kind of food ___________________________________

____

Appetite: Poor Average Good

Slept from _______ to ________ Total: ______

Felt rested after waking: Yes No

Side Effects: ___________________________________

____

____

____

____

Symptom Details

Rate the following on a scale of 1 to 5:
(1-Poor 2- Meh 3- Decent 4- Good 5-Super)

Mood _____ Focus _____ Memory _____

Energy _____ Motivation _____ Finishing Tasks _____

Patience _____ Impulsivity _____ Restlessness _____

Time Management _____ Emotion Management _____

Other: _______________ _____ _________________ ____

Medication helped today: Yes No Somewhat

Today's Successes: ________________________________

____

____

____

____

Areas for Improvement: ___________________________

____

____

____

Rating for This Day
1- Awful / 5- Great

☆☆☆☆☆

Medication Details

Date ____________ ____________ Day of Week

Medication ____________ Dosage __________

Skipped Medication Yes No

Time(s) medication taken:

AM __________ AM __________
PM __________ PM __________

Time(s) medication wore off: ________ ________

Taken: [1] [2] On empty stomach
[1] [2] With Food

Kind of food __________________________________

____

Appetite: Poor Average Good

Slept from ________ to _________ Total: _______

Felt rested after waking: Yes No

Side Effects: ___________________________________

____

____

____

____

Symptom Details

Rate the following on a scale of 1 to 5:
(1-Poor 2- Meh 3- Decent 4- Good 5-Super)

Mood _____ Focus _____ Memory _____

Energy _____ Motivation _____ Finishing Tasks _____

Patience _____ Impulsivity _____ Restlessness _____

Time Management _____ Emotion Management _____

Other: _______________ _____ _________________ ____

Medication helped today: Yes No Somewhat

Today's Successes: ______________________________

____

____

____

____

Areas for Improvement: ________________________

____

____

____

Rating for This Day
1- Awful / 5- Great

☆☆☆☆☆

Medication Details

Date ______________ ______________ Day of Week

Medication ______________ Dosage ___________

Skipped Medication Yes No

Time(s) medication taken:

AM ___________ AM ___________
PM ___________ PM ___________

Time(s) medication wore off: _________ _________

Taken: [1] [2] On empty stomach
[1] [2] With Food

Kind of food _______________________________________

____

Appetite: Poor Average Good

Slept from _________ to __________ Total: _______

Felt rested after waking: Yes No

Side Effects: ____

____

____

____

____

Symptom Details

Rate the following on a scale of 1 to 5:
(1-Poor 2- Meh 3- Decent 4- Good 5-Super)

Mood _____ Focus _____ Memory _____

Energy _____ Motivation _____ Finishing Tasks _____

Patience _____ Impulsivity _____ Restlessness _____

Time Management _____ Emotion Management _____

Other: ______________ _____ ________________ ____

Medication helped today: Yes No Somewhat

Today's Successes: ________________________________

____

____

____

____

Areas for Improvement: __________________________

____

____

____

Rating for This Day
1- Awful / 5- Great

☆☆☆☆☆

Medication Details

Date _______________ _______________ Day of Week

Medication _______________ Dosage ____________

Skipped Medication Yes No

Time(s) medication taken:

AM ____________ AM ____________
PM ____________ PM ____________

Time(s) medication wore off: _________ _________

Taken: [1] [2] On empty stomach
[1] [2] With Food

Kind of food ____

____

Appetite: Poor Average Good

Slept from _________ to ___________ Total: ________

Felt rested after waking: Yes No

Side Effects: ____

____

____

____

____

Symptom Details

Rate the following on a scale of 1 to 5:
(1-Poor 2- Meh 3- Decent 4- Good 5-Super)

Mood _____ Focus _____ Memory _____

Energy _____ Motivation _____ Finishing Tasks _____

Patience _____ Impulsivity _____ Restlessness _____

Time Management _____ Emotion Management _____

Other: ________________ _____ __________________ ____

Medication helped today: Yes No Somewhat

Today's Successes: ____________________________________

____

____

____

____

Areas for Improvement: ____________________________

____

____

____

Rating for This Day
1- Awful / 5- Great

☆☆☆☆☆

Medication Details

Date ____________ ____________ Day of Week

Medication ____________ Dosage __________

Skipped Medication Yes No

Time(s) medication taken:

AM __________ AM __________
PM __________ PM __________

Time(s) medication wore off: ________ ________

Taken: [1] [2] On empty stomach
[1] [2] With Food

Kind of food ____________________________________

____

Appetite: Poor Average Good

Slept from ________ to ________ Total: ______

Felt rested after waking: Yes No

Side Effects: ____________________________________

____

____

____

____

Symptom Details

Rate the following on a scale of 1 to 5:
(1-Poor 2- Meh 3- Decent 4- Good 5-Super)

Mood _____ Focus _____ Memory _____

Energy _____ Motivation _____ Finishing Tasks _____

Patience _____ Impulsivity _____ Restlessness _____

Time Management _____ Emotion Management _____

Other: _______________ _____ _______________ _____

Medication helped today: Yes No Somewhat

Today's Successes: ______________________________

____

____

____

____

Areas for Improvement: ______________________________

____

____

____

Rating for This Day
1- Awful / 5- Great

☆☆☆☆☆

Medication Details

Date ______________ ______________ Day of Week

Medication ______________ Dosage ___________

Skipped Medication Yes No

Time(s) medication taken:

AM ___________ AM ___________
PM ___________ PM ___________

Time(s) medication wore off: ________ ________

Taken: ☐1 ☐2 On empty stomach
☐1 ☐2 With Food

Kind of food ____

____

Appetite: Poor Average Good

Slept from ________ to _________ Total: _______

Felt rested after waking: Yes No

Side Effects: ____

____

____

____

____

Symptom Details

Rate the following on a scale of 1 to 5:
(1-Poor 2- Meh 3- Decent 4- Good 5-Super)

Mood _____ Focus _____ Memory _____

Energy _____ Motivation _____ Finishing Tasks _____

Patience _____ Impulsivity _____ Restlessness _____

Time Management _____ Emotion Management _____

Other: _______________ _____ _________________ ____

Medication helped today: Yes No Somewhat

Today's Successes: __________________________________

____

____

____

____

Areas for Improvement: ____________________________

____

____

____

Rating for This Day
1- Awful / 5- Great

☆☆☆☆☆

Medication Details

Date ______________ ______________ Day of Week

Medication ______________ Dosage ___________

Skipped Medication Yes No

Time(s) medication taken:

AM ___________ AM ___________
PM ___________ PM ___________

Time(s) medication wore off: ________ ________

Taken: [1] [2] On empty stomach
[1] [2] With Food

Kind of food ______________________________________

____

Appetite: Poor Average Good

Slept from ________ to __________ Total: _______

Felt rested after waking: Yes No

Side Effects: ______________________________________

____

____

____

____

Symptom Details

Rate the following on a scale of 1 to 5:
(1-Poor 2- Meh 3- Decent 4- Good 5-Super)

Mood _____ Focus _____ Memory _____

Energy _____ Motivation _____ Finishing Tasks _____

Patience _____ Impulsivity _____ Restlessness _____

Time Management _____ Emotion Management _____

Other: _______________ _____ _______________ ____

Medication helped today: Yes No Somewhat

Today's Successes: ______________________________

____

____

____

____

Areas for Improvement: __________________________

____

____

____

Rating for This Day
1- Awful / 5- Great

☆☆☆☆☆

Medication Details

Date ____________ ____________ Day of Week

Medication ____________ Dosage __________

Skipped Medication Yes No

Time(s) medication taken:

AM __________ AM __________
PM __________ PM __________

Time(s) medication wore off: ________ ________

Taken: [1] [2] On empty stomach
[1] [2] With Food

Kind of food ____________________________________

____

Appetite: Poor Average Good

Slept from ________ to _________ Total: _______

Felt rested after waking: Yes No

Side Effects: ____________________________________

____

____

____

____

Symptom Details

Rate the following on a scale of 1 to 5:
(1-Poor 2- Meh 3- Decent 4- Good 5-Super)

Mood _____ Focus _____ Memory _____

Energy _____ Motivation _____ Finishing Tasks _____

Patience _____ Impulsivity _____ Restlessness _____

Time Management _____ Emotion Management _____

Other: ______________ _____ ________________ ____

Medication helped today: Yes No Somewhat

Today's Successes: ________________________________

____

____

____

____

Areas for Improvement: __________________________

____

____

____

Rating for This Day
1- Awful / 5- Great

☆☆☆☆☆

Medication Details

Date ____________ ____________ Day of Week

Medication ____________ Dosage __________

Skipped Medication Yes No

Time(s) medication taken:

AM __________ AM __________
PM __________ PM __________

Time(s) medication wore off: ________ ________

Taken: [1] [2] On empty stomach
[1] [2] With Food

Kind of food ______________________________

____

Appetite: Poor Average Good

Slept from ________ to _________ Total: _______

Felt rested after waking: Yes No

Side Effects: ______________________________

____

____

____

____

Symptom Details

Rate the following on a scale of 1 to 5:
(1-Poor 2- Meh 3- Decent 4- Good 5-Super)

Mood _____ Focus _____ Memory _____

Energy _____ Motivation _____ Finishing Tasks _____

Patience _____ Impulsivity _____ Restlessness _____

Time Management _____ Emotion Management _____

Other: ______________ _____ ________________ ____

Medication helped today: Yes No Somewhat

Today's Successes: ________________________________

____

____

____

____

Areas for Improvement: __________________________

____

____

____

Rating for This Day
1- Awful / 5- Great

☆☆☆☆☆

Medication Details

Date ____________ ____________ Day of Week

Medication ____________ Dosage __________

Skipped Medication Yes No

Time(s) medication taken:

AM __________ AM __________
PM __________ PM __________

Time(s) medication wore off: ________ ________

Taken: [1] [2] On empty stomach
[1] [2] With Food

Kind of food ___________________________________

____

Appetite: Poor Average Good

Slept from ________ to _________ Total: _______

Felt rested after waking: Yes No

Side Effects: ___________________________________

____

____

____

____

Symptom Details

Rate the following on a scale of 1 to 5:
(1-Poor 2- Meh 3- Decent 4- Good 5-Super)

Mood _____ Focus _____ Memory _____

Energy _____ Motivation _____ Finishing Tasks _____

Patience _____ Impulsivity _____ Restlessness _____

Time Management _____ Emotion Management _____

Other: ______________ _____ ______________ ____

Medication helped today: Yes No Somewhat

Today's Successes: ______________________________

____

____

____

____

Areas for Improvement: ___________________________

____

____

____

Rating for This Day
1- Awful / 5- Great

☆☆☆☆☆

Medication Details

Date ____________ ____________ Day of Week

Medication ____________ Dosage __________

Skipped Medication Yes No

Time(s) medication taken:

AM __________ AM __________
PM __________ PM __________

Time(s) medication wore off: ________ ________

Taken: [1] [2] On empty stomach
[1] [2] With Food

Kind of food ____________________________________

____

Appetite: Poor Average Good

Slept from ________ to _________ Total: _______

Felt rested after waking: Yes No

Side Effects: ____________________________________

____

____

____

____

Symptom Details

Rate the following on a scale of 1 to 5:
(1-Poor 2- Meh 3- Decent 4- Good 5-Super)

Mood _____ Focus _____ Memory _____

Energy _____ Motivation _____ Finishing Tasks _____

Patience _____ Impulsivity _____ Restlessness _____

Time Management _____ Emotion Management _____

Other: ______________ _____ ______________ ____

Medication helped today: Yes No Somewhat

Today's Successes: ______________________________

____

____

____

____

Areas for Improvement: __________________________

____

____

____

Rating for This Day
1- Awful / 5- Great

☆☆☆☆☆

Medication Details

Date ____________ ____________ Day of Week

Medication ____________ Dosage __________

Skipped Medication Yes No

Time(s) medication taken:

AM __________ AM __________
PM __________ PM __________

Time(s) medication wore off: ________ ________

Taken: ☐1 ☐2 On empty stomach
☐1 ☐2 With Food

Kind of food ____________________________________

____

Appetite: Poor Average Good

Slept from ________ to _________ Total: _______

Felt rested after waking: Yes No

Side Effects: ___________________________________

____

____

____

____

Symptom Details

Rate the following on a scale of 1 to 5:
(1-Poor 2- Meh 3- Decent 4- Good 5-Super)

Mood _____ Focus _____ Memory _____

Energy _____ Motivation _____ Finishing Tasks _____

Patience _____ Impulsivity _____ Restlessness _____

Time Management _____ Emotion Management _____

Other: _______________ _____ _________________ ____

Medication helped today: Yes No Somewhat

Today's Successes: ________________________________

____

____

____

____

Areas for Improvement: ___________________________

____

____

____

Rating for This Day
1- Awful / 5- Great

☆☆☆☆☆

Medication Details

Date ____________ ____________ Day of Week

Medication ____________ Dosage __________

Skipped Medication Yes No

Time(s) medication taken:

AM __________ AM __________
PM __________ PM __________

Time(s) medication wore off: ________ ________

Taken: [1] [2] On empty stomach
[1] [2] With Food

Kind of food ______________________________________

____

Appetite: Poor Average Good

Slept from ________ to _________ Total: _______

Felt rested after waking: Yes No

Side Effects: ____________________________________

____

____

____

____

Symptom Details

Rate the following on a scale of 1 to 5:
(1-Poor 2- Meh 3- Decent 4- Good 5-Super)

Mood _____ Focus _____ Memory _____

Energy _____ Motivation _____ Finishing Tasks _____

Patience _____ Impulsivity _____ Restlessness _____

Time Management _____ Emotion Management _____

Other: _______________ _____ _______________ ____

Medication helped today: Yes No Somewhat

Today's Successes: ______________________________

____

____

____

____

Areas for Improvement: __________________________

____

____

____

Rating for This Day
1- Awful / 5- Great

☆☆☆☆☆

Medication Details

Date ____________ ____________ Day of Week

Medication ____________ Dosage __________

Skipped Medication Yes No

Time(s) medication taken:

AM __________ AM __________
PM __________ PM __________

Time(s) medication wore off: _______ _______

Taken: [1] [2] On empty stomach
[1] [2] With Food

Kind of food __________________________________

____

Appetite: Poor Average Good

Slept from _______ to ________ Total: ______

Felt rested after waking: Yes No

Side Effects: __________________________________

____

____

____

____

Symptom Details

Rate the following on a scale of 1 to 5:
(1-Poor 2- Meh 3- Decent 4- Good 5-Super)

Mood _____ Focus _____ Memory _____

Energy _____ Motivation _____ Finishing Tasks _____

Patience _____ Impulsivity _____ Restlessness _____

Time Management _____ Emotion Management _____

Other: _______________ _____ _________________ ____

Medication helped today: Yes No Somewhat

Today's Successes: __________________________________

____

____

____

____

Areas for Improvement: ____________________________

____

____

____

Rating for This Day
1- Awful / 5- Great

☆☆☆☆☆

Medication Details

Date ____________ ____________ Day of Week

Medication ____________ Dosage __________

Skipped Medication Yes No

Time(s) medication taken:

AM __________ AM __________
PM __________ PM __________

Time(s) medication wore off: ________ ________

Taken: ☐1 ☐2 On empty stomach
☐1 ☐2 With Food

Kind of food ______________________________________

____

Appetite: Poor Average Good

Slept from ________ to _________ Total: ______

Felt rested after waking: Yes No

Side Effects: ____________________________________

____

____

____

____

Symptom Details

Rate the following on a scale of 1 to 5:
(1-Poor 2- Meh 3- Decent 4- Good 5-Super)

Mood _____ Focus _____ Memory _____

Energy _____ Motivation _____ Finishing Tasks _____

Patience _____ Impulsivity _____ Restlessness _____

Time Management _____ Emotion Management _____

Other: _______________ _____ _________________ ____

Medication helped today: Yes No Somewhat

Today's Successes: __________________________________

____

____

____

____

Areas for Improvement: ____________________________

____

____

____

Rating for This Day
1- Awful / 5- Great

☆☆☆☆☆

Medication Details

Date ____________ ____________ Day of Week

Medication ____________ Dosage __________

Skipped Medication Yes No

Time(s) medication taken:

AM __________ AM __________
PM __________ PM __________

Time(s) medication wore off: _______ _______

Taken: ☐1 ☐2 On empty stomach
☐1 ☐2 With Food

Kind of food __________________________________

____

Appetite: Poor Average Good

Slept from _______ to ________ Total: ______

Felt rested after waking: Yes No

Side Effects: ___________________________________

____

____

____

____

Symptom Details

Rate the following on a scale of 1 to 5:
(1-Poor 2- Meh 3- Decent 4- Good 5-Super)

Mood _____ Focus _____ Memory _____

Energy _____ Motivation _____ Finishing Tasks _____

Patience _____ Impulsivity _____ Restlessness _____

Time Management _____ Emotion Management _____

Other: ______________ _____ ________________ ____

Medication helped today: Yes No Somewhat

Today's Successes: ________________________________

____

____

____

____

Areas for Improvement: __________________________

____

____

____

Rating for This Day
1- Awful / 5- Great

☆☆☆☆☆

Medication Details

Date ____________ ____________ Day of Week

Medication ____________ Dosage __________

Skipped Medication Yes No

Time(s) medication taken:

AM __________ AM __________
PM __________ PM __________

Time(s) medication wore off: ________ ________

Taken: [1] [2] On empty stomach
[1] [2] With Food

Kind of food ____

____

Appetite: Poor Average Good

Slept from ________ to _________ Total: _______

Felt rested after waking: Yes No

Side Effects: ____

____

____

____

____

Symptom Details

Rate the following on a scale of 1 to 5:
(1-Poor 2- Meh 3- Decent 4- Good 5-Super)

Mood _____ Focus _____ Memory _____

Energy _____ Motivation _____ Finishing Tasks _____

Patience _____ Impulsivity _____ Restlessness _____

Time Management _____ Emotion Management _____

Other: ________________ _____ ________________ ____

Medication helped today: Yes No Somewhat

Today's Successes: ________________________________

____

____

____

____

Areas for Improvement: ____________________________

____

____

____

Rating for This Day
1- Awful / 5- Great

☆☆☆☆☆

Medication Details

Date ____________ ____________ Day of Week

Medication ____________ Dosage __________

Skipped Medication Yes No

Time(s) medication taken:

AM __________ AM __________
PM __________ PM __________

Time(s) medication wore off: ________ ________

Taken: ☐1 ☐2 On empty stomach
☐1 ☐2 With Food

Kind of food ___________________________________

____

Appetite: Poor Average Good

Slept from ________ to _________ Total: _______

Felt rested after waking: Yes No

Side Effects: ___________________________________

____

____

____

____

Symptom Details

Rate the following on a scale of 1 to 5:
(1-Poor 2- Meh 3- Decent 4- Good 5-Super)

Mood _____ Focus _____ Memory _____

Energy _____ Motivation _____ Finishing Tasks _____

Patience _____ Impulsivity _____ Restlessness _____

Time Management _____ Emotion Management _____

Other: _______________ _____ _______________ ____

Medication helped today: Yes No Somewhat

Today's Successes: ______________________________

____

____

____

____

Areas for Improvement: __________________________

____

____

____

Rating for This Day
1- Awful / 5- Great

☆☆☆☆☆

Medication Details

Date ____________ ____________ Day of Week

Medication ____________ Dosage __________

Skipped Medication Yes No

Time(s) medication taken:

AM __________ AM __________
PM __________ PM __________

Time(s) medication wore off: ________ ________

Taken: ☐1 ☐2 On empty stomach
☐1 ☐2 With Food

Kind of food ______________________________

____

Appetite: Poor Average Good

Slept from ________ to ________ Total: ______

Felt rested after waking: Yes No

Side Effects: ______________________________

____

____

____

____

Symptom Details

Rate the following on a scale of 1 to 5:
(1-Poor 2- Meh 3- Decent 4- Good 5-Super)

Mood _____ Focus _____ Memory _____

Energy _____ Motivation _____ Finishing Tasks _____

Patience _____ Impulsivity _____ Restlessness _____

Time Management _____ Emotion Management _____

Other: _______________ _____ _______________ ____

Medication helped today: Yes No Somewhat

Today's Successes: ______________________________

____

____

____

____

Areas for Improvement: __________________________

____

____

____

Rating for This Day
1- Awful / 5- Great

☆☆☆☆☆

Made in the USA
Monee, IL
04 November 2026

67375695R00108